STAY FOCUS! STAY HEALTY

Lose Your Weight by Changing Your Mind

Marygrace Sun

TABLE OF CONTENTS

CHAPTER ONE
GETTING STARTED WITH WEIGHT LOSS

Understanding Weight Loss

It is true that every problem has a solution which is not part of the problem itself. Therefore, before you can proffer a solution to any problem, you must first identify what that problem is. In other words, before anybody can proffer solutions on how to lose weight, there must be a certified causes of your weight gain. Some of the notable questions that people who want to shed some weight frequently ask are:

How do people get to this point that weight becomes a problem?

What causes weight gain?

Why is it easier to gain weight than to lose weight?

When these questions have been fully settled, then, we can talk about the remedies to weight loss?'

It is easier to gain weight but difficult to lose weight which shows that weight loss is not a day's job. To lose weight, there are some key factors that must be established in your mind and these factors are:

Realizing your need to shed off some weight and get your confidence back.

Be willingly to make sacrifices that will enhance your weight loss no matter the cost.

You must understand Time Management is important in weight loss journey.

Diet has everything to do with Weight loss. Patience and Consistency is a key element to imbibe as a lifestyle if you must achieve your weight loss goal. Losing weight naturally is the most effective and healthy way. It involves a better diet, an exercise which amounts to a better lifestyle. Losing weight is a life style you have to learn and gradually live by it. Losing weight naturally does not mean you should forbid certain foods but that you should eat healthier ingredients than usual. So, don't push yourself so hard to adopt but gradually accept to make changes till you can completely eliminate those items that causes weight gain.

Please note that, there is no magical diet that or slimming down recipe or tea or fat burning scheme that is going to wipe away weight gain and keep those pounds away once you're done with them. Avoid all these quick weight loss schemes promising you a quick reshape within a short time because there is nothing like that and in the long run, you will end up gaining a weight than before because the rules and regulations are difficult to maintain and you end up damaging your body system. Thus, losing weight naturally is better for your overall health and it will last in the long run. Never forget that true healthy weight loss requires a Lifestyle change and Hardworking! When it comes to weight loss, many already missed it from their focus and that's why they're finding it frustrating achieving their desired weight.

So, how do you start releasing yourself of this frustration and achieving your desired weight as fast as you desire? First thing first, channel your energies appropriately and redirect your focus.

When you set out and tell yourself 'I want to lose

weight' then you get more of the weight or you find it difficult to follow through on the process to the weight you desire.

Losing weight is never the problem, how you see your weight is the problem.

And if you can change how you see any experience then you start changing the experience. What the help of suitable friends and teammates, you can get those quick results that you've always desired

So instead of killing yourself...

'I want to lose weight' or 'How do I lose this my weight?' and allowing all those weight loss programs or products to continue to swallow your money unnecessarily.

(This does not mean that they don't work)

You may have read almost everything you can on weight loss and seems as though there's nothing new anymore. But then, it is still pertinent that you open up spaces for some other knowledge and findings.

You see, many people rush into weight loss programs and rush out again. Below are some of the following tips which if you follow will help you in your journey.

- **Admit That You Have a Bad Shape**

Against the backdrop of whatever kind of shape or weight you want. Admit your presence shape/weight and know it's not a fault.

See, you must understand, that there is nothing like right or perfect weight. Those are the gimmicks of those weight management companies and entertainment/fashion industries to sell to you.

Just as lots of people like it portable, some like it light and some like it loaded...individual with his preference.

You'll agree with me that your weight is your weight until that moment by somehow means something somehow initiated your desire for a different form or shape. Now, ask yourself is this decision truly yours or some sort of people-pleasing gimmicks on your mind.

In all, the place to start is to first admit your present weight/shape.

- **Have a Mental Picture of Your Ideal Shape**

What Pounds or Kilograms Would You Want to Weigh?

Stop this disempowering attitude of comparing yourself to someone else. 'If I can just lose this weight and be like Brenda or Lolita, I would be better off.' The raw fact is, you can't be like those people you want to be like and that's what is actually frustrating you.

This is you. This is your life. The moment you start the game of comparison you relinquish your power of confidence in yourself and you lose the game. And you put yourself under pressure and you begin to find the process not producing the result you want. Because day by day you want to look in the mirror and see Brenda or Lolita and they're nowhere to be found.

Focus on the pounds, not your friends.

- **Summon Your Determinative Energy and Self-Will**

Assuming your desire weight is more of your self-will and self-discipline, you are truly not going to have that ideal weight and size that you desire. If you truly will it you will find a way to it. The level of your self-will towards your desire weight will help you generate the required self-discipline.

Many dropped along the way from the gym program that they signed up for because they have no enough self-will towards that pounds/kg they desire.

- **Create An Environment That Facilitates What You Want**

Alexander Den Heijer said, "When a flower doesn't bloom, you fix the environment in which it grows, not the flower.

Your environment in this context includes your food, your circle of influence, your TV/radio programs, and your apartment arrangement.

You have to make them align to help you achieve your weight goal faster.

- **Live the Very Change You Desire**

Act in your desired weight. Do the things your desire weight will do.

Go ahead and decide the weight loss process that suits

you...and be sure you enjoy the process. In the enjoyment of your weight loss process lies the speed to your desired weight.

If you are not very sure of what to do, kindly ask your weight management coach about the process that suits you.

Have a Good Reason

People go into weight loss sometimes for the wrong reasons, sometimes just because people say you're fat or your clothes no longer fit and some other reasons that really don't hold water. I'm listing a few reasons you should consider losing weight:

- **Are You Overweight?**

Being overweight cannot be determined by just looking at yourself in the mirror. A singular parameter is used in judging whether you're overweight, underweight or obese that is the Body Mass Index (BMI).

Okay, this involves a little Math.

Your Body mass index is the ratio of your Weight (Body Mass) to the square of your height. So you can calculate your BMI right away: just divide your current body weight with the square of your height and you have your BMI.

A body mass of below 18.5 is considered underweight, 18.5 - 24.9 is normal or healthy, once you hit 25 mark, boom!!! You are overweight, anything above 30 is considered obesity.

- **Are You Losing Your Confidence?**

When you start losing your confidence because of how you look, you should consider losing weight (as much as your looks shouldn't be a major determinant of who you are, you know when you're no longer confident in your own skin, and since it's a situation that can be changed, you could consider going for the better change). A beautiful thing about this is that it's a morale booster because when you decide to do something and then you achieve it, it increases your faith in yourself.

What are Your Weight Loss Targets?

Set targets for yourself. How many Kilograms or Pounds of weight do you intend losing? And how long do you want to take? This will keep you in track and help you monitor your progress. For instance if you intend to lose 12 kilograms in one month, you should break it down into four weeks and try to lose 3 kilograms weekly. In setting your target you should apply the SMART principle of goal setting: specific, measurable, achievable, realistic and time bound.

- **Be Patient with Yourself**

The weight didn't jump on you, it happened over a period of time so as you start your journey allow yourself enjoy the process. Just ensure you make steady daily progress.

Weight loss usually happens at a rate of 0.5-1kg (1-2lbs) a week so if you've got a big weight loss goal, then you need to chip away at it, one week at a time.

It can take you weeks or months to get to where you desire to be. With consistency, you can even lose 56 pounds (25kg) in just 6 months. Then you achieve this tiny goal of yours, you would be ecstatic to be able to get this far after all the time and efforts you are sacrificing.

"You do not add all those weight in one day; and you certainly would not lose it one day. You have to be patient to get best results."

When this starts happening, just know that you are still in a journey. You still have about one hand luggage size of weight to shed off. When you fully get to your goal weight, you will surely hire a photographer and commemorate this once in a lifetime achievement with some professional Photo-shoots.

Same for running a business. There is no overnight success in business. That successful business person you see today has spent a lot of time behind the scenes setting up their own stage. Yet, they still work hard because with success comes more responsibility and opportunity for even more success.

The truth is Rapid results are not always sustainable. Remember to reward yourself for small successes along the way too.

- **Talk About It**

Life and death are in the power of the tongue. So let people around you know you're trying to achieve a goal.

Also by saying it, you're reminding your body that you are trying to achieve something here. And you know what? Your body listens.

- **Understand Weight Loss**

Wisdom is the principal thing, in all and in all your getting, get understanding. When you understood how weight loss works, it became a lot easier to give up some kind of food and take up on some kind of activities. This is what you would normally not do. So read up everything you can, understand your body, calories, food portioning and how weight loss works.

Useful Lessons You can learn during Your Weight Loss Journey

Weight Loss is something that most people want but will rarely achieve in their lifetime. Some people have always wanted to lose weight when they detect that they are weighing more than normal but the drive and the persistence to continue always falls short and hence, they were never able get started.

Losing weight is easily one of the hardest things that can you can ever try achieving, it requires an outrageous amount of discipline and mental strength as well. In fact, many people who have lost weight have recounted how they have immensely benefitted from their decisions, of course not without tales of the tiring days that had to endure. Below Are Five Major Lessons That You Can Learn In Your Journey to Weight Loss:

- **You Must Put In the Required Amount of Work**

When you first start your weight loss journey, it is sure that you would be desperately hoping that there was some special "miracle pill" that you could take for a few weeks and then magically have a toned body.

Most people start their journey started out by looking for the "quick solution" and the easy way out. But as we all know, there's no magic pill to sustainable weight loss. There's no miracle pill to making starting and growing your business either. You've got to put in the work.

- **Consult the Services of Your Friends or Teammates and Follow Their Advice When Necessary**

So fine. After coming to the conclusion that you needed to put forth some real effort into losing weight, you will have to start making attempts at eating healthy and exercising. Do not eat supposedly healthy foods that are labelled low-fat. This is because they are dangerous to your body. A lot of those low-fat labelled food out there have some many hidden sugars and other non-healthy substitutes added. You would be making things worse for yourself if you indulge in the habit of consuming such foods.

Some weight loss enthusiasts have ended up spending all of their efforts on eating the wrong way because they had no clue what the heck they are doing. In reality, they should have known better Just like with starting a business, it's really easy to jump right in and waste a ton of time doing stuff that doesn't matter. If you want to make progress quickly, you need to consult with someone that knows what they are doing and learn from them.

- **Find Out What Works Best For You**

A lot of weight loss enthusiasts have consulted with several people who had successfully achieved weight loss status. They heard of different weight loss diets and supplements such as Clean 9, noodles diet, juicing, milkshake, Lemon and ginger, Cambridge diet, etc. It is interesting to know there are so many diets out there – What a huge industry!

You may like something natural – no pills, no concocted drinks, and no processed meals. Also, something affordable may appeal to you. If this is you, try devising your own plan that was specifically tailored to your personality. You can also try out the Ketogenic Lifestyle albeit customized to suit your weight loss goals, your own lifestyle and your personality. You can deal with it.

You can get as much advice as you want from experts or business gurus, but when it comes down to it, every business and/or diet is going to be different. At some point, you will have to take what you have learned and tailor things to your own situation. And only you will know what is best for yourself.

- **It Is More Fun-Filled When You Do It with Your Friend And Teammates**

Losing weight is hard work and it's good to know that others are going through a similar battle. It's also good to be able to talk to other like-minded people who are equally ensconced in meal plans, kilograms lost and body measurements!

In the same way that support groups and personal trainers help people to lose weight, networking groups, coaches and mentors do the same for business. Having people you can share your woes and successes with, go to for help when you get stuck, learn new techniques from and who keep you accountable will greatly increases your chance of business success.

What lessons from areas of your life can you apply to running your business?

Three Pitfalls to Avoid for you to be Successful on your Weight Loss Journey

1. Stop Looking For Quick Fixes or Shortcuts

After one or two weeks of following a program some people wants to have lost all the weight they gained in years. It doesn't work that way, you have to give it time because you didn't gain the weight in one day.

The work starts from inside your body. A lot of cleansing of all the unhealthy food you have been feeding your body for years have to take place first after which your body will start using up the fat stored in your glycogen store in your body.

When the store is exhausted then you will start losing weight and see physical evidence.

2. Not Following Your Meal Plan

Don't eat outside your meal, eat what you're asked to eat for effective results

There are reasons why some particular foods are on your meal plan and some are not.

Trust your coach because they know what they are doing except otherwise.

Eating outside your meal plan stalls your progress.

Ask for substitutes if you can't get or afford some of the items on your plan.

3. Not Exercising

Part of the reason why you're overweight in the first place is because you're living a life of inactivity.

CHAPTER TWO
EXERCISE AND WEIGHT LOSS

The Man Who Lost 90 Pounds with the Help of His Girlfriend

Jared found out early enough that he is among those who are inclined to sports. And it was no question if he was fit then. But unfortunately, the 27-years old Jared gained appreciable weight when he found himself in a relationship, courtesy to the relative sedentary lifestyle that he was living. With his girlfriend Samantha MacDonald, they'll spend all nights snacking so that in no time, he gained a whopping 285 lb. But then, he had a quick realization. He must do something about his health and body size if he have to enjoy the lifestyle and physique that he often crave for. His resolve even became stronger when he opened his refrigerator one day and saw all manner of pizza boxes. He decided that his eating habits is going to change from that day.

"To say the least, it is awkward, but that is the truth," Jared told CNN. "When I open the refrigerator, I was just like, 'What that hell do we have here?'"

Jared and his girlfriend made the decision of trying out intermittent fasting. They made it a habit to eat their meals between noon and 8 p.m. What they instantly noticed was stunning. They discovered that they have increased energy levels, plus their drive to become more active also increased. When they saw the amazing results that is yielded, they practiced indoor cycling for 45 minutes every six days in a week.

"We were helpful to one another in strengthening our weak areas," MacDonald said. "Initially, we were on different levels but we later realized the importance of being on the same page and we pushed for it. We were not wrong because the result was a huge success."

In about seven months, Jared was able to shed off 95 pounds. He is currently a fitness instructor when he teach his student about indoor cycling. MacDonald on the other hand was able to shed 12 pounds. According to her, the real win is the mental benefit that she derive in going to the gym every day and sticking with it.

"It was enormously advantageous to have a system of support with me," he said. "The truth is that, every day is unique and each comes with its own temptation. Sometimes you'll want to convince yourself to take a bite of the pizza when your partner is not watching. But the mere fact that there is a support system to help you check your excesses and balances and also being responsible for your actions was helpful in making sure that I don't cross my boundary."

Exercising Your Way to Health

When it comes to living the best of life, the place of a quality exercise cannot be overlooked, but many have overlooked it and that is why the rate of illness and obesity increases daily.

Follow your exercise routine; it works with your meal plan to help you burn more calories. Also note that unless you are in a calorie deficit every day, you will not lose weight.

Calories are less than calories = weight loss

Exercise also helps boost your metabolism. It starts or wakes up your system for optimal operation.

Exercise has a lot of health advantages and this is how you will benefit from it.

Here are the advantages of regular exercise.

- Exercise Weight Controls

Exercise can help reduce unnecessary weight gain, or help sustain weight loss. You burn calories while you're involved in physical activity. The exercise gets more intense, the more calories you burn.

Daily gym trips are fine, but don't panic if you can't find a large chunk of time every day to workout. Any amount of operation is better than absolutely zero.

Just get more involved in the day to reap the benefits of exercise — take the stairs instead of the elevator, or revive the household chores. Consistency is essential.

- Exercise Combats Health Conditions And Diseases

Are you worried about gaining weight?

No matter what your current weight is, being active boosts high-density lipoprotein (HDL) cholesterol, the "good" cholesterol, and it decreases unhealthy triglycerides.

This one-two punch keeps your blood flowing smoothly, which decreases your risk of cardiovascular diseases.

Regular exercise helps manage or prevent many health concerns and problems, such as High blood pressure, Metabolic syndrome, Stroke, Anxiety, Depression, Type 2 diabetes, Arthritis, and Many types of cancer.

It may also help enhance cognitive function and help to reduce the likelihood of all causes of death.

- Improves Mood

Need a mental lift? And will they need to let off some steam after a day of stress?

A brisk walk or a gym session may help. Physical exercise activates different chemicals in the brain which can make you feel happy, more comfortable and less nervous.

Often, when you exercise regularly you can feel better about your appearance and yourself, which can boost your morale and increase your self-esteem.

- Exercise Boosts Energy

Daily physical activity will enhance your muscle stre ngth and increase your stamina. Exercise supplies the bo dy with oxygen and nutrients, and improves the cardiova scular health

And when your heart and lung health improve, you have more energy to tackle daily chores.

"If you have determination, drive, and discipline … nothing is impossible."

- **Exercise Can Be Social … And Fun!**

Exercise and physical activity can be enjoyable.

They give you a chance to unwind, enjoy the outdoors or simply engage in activities that make you happy. Physical activity can also help you connect with family or friends in a fun social setting. So take a dance class, hit the hiking trails or join a soccer team. Find a physical activity you enjoy, and just do it. Bored? Try something new, or do something with friends or family. Exercise and physical activity are great ways to feel better, boost your health and have fun.

For most healthy adults, the many fitness outlets and nutritionists jointly recommends:

At least 150 minutes a week of moderate aerobic exercise, or 75 minutes a week of intense aerobic activity, or a mix of moderate activity and vigor.

The recommendations recommend you spread the workout all week long.

Examples include biking, running or swimming. Only small amounts of physical activity are beneficial, and cumulative day-round exercise adds up to the health benefits.

Strength training drills, at least two days a week, for all major muscle groups. Types include free weight lifting, weight machine use or body weight exercise.

Disseminate your tasks during the week. If you want to lose weight, reach clear exercise goals, you can need to scale up your moderate aerobic exercise to more than 300 minutes a week.

Before beginning a new exercise plan, remember to consult with your doctor, particularly if you have questions about your fitness, have not been exercising for a long time, has chronic health issues including heart disease and diabetes.

Know wellbeing is the most precious asset. Safety secures it as a priceless gift.

Popular Reasons That Keep People From Exercising

For everyone who's ever tried to sustain a fitness routine to build muscles, lose weight or burn belly fats, build six packs, there are reasons, so familiar to us what we make to feel good about.

You are aware that the program is good

You are aware that you took it up by yourself after reading some nice article or, seeing someone you love looking good because of their workout programs.

You are also aware that you needed this and that it will help you to get in shape as you have always wanted and dreamed about but……YOU ARE JUST NOT DOING IT

Why?

Well, below are just 5 common reasons we usually give for skipping our weight loss exercises.

And we actually manufacture these excuses just to make ourselves feel less guilt for not achieving a certain goal we set for ourselves.

- **I Have Tried This Before**

Discouragement is real. No one likes failures and no likes to fail. Sometimes, it saps our energy and makes us feel like we just cannot get it right. Set goals that are small and realistic.

Then you're more likely to feel like a success, not a failure. It also helps to keep a log and post it somewhere public -- even on Facebook.

You can post what you are up to so that your friends can hold you accountable.

Of course, you will have to post again how far you got. This simple act can help you keep to something.

- **I Am Too Tired**

When you are feeling tired or just feeling like not getting up and doing something in the house, it will frequently work for you when you do some exercises like squats.

Some press ups or push-ups would get me into the powerful mood again and seem to have borrowed energy from some store.

"Have a particular time for it. Stick it out and get it done. Nobody ever got strong or got in shape by thinking about it. They did it."

Try it and stop giving excuses. So, it actually follows that exercising actually boosts your energy because it gives out that endorphins or "feel good" hormones too.

Of course you are tired, who isn't? Believe it or not, exercise actually boosts your energy levels.

If you are too tired after work, try going before work, even if it means getting up when it's still dark out.

Just make sure you have an exercise plan so that you don't walk around the gym half asleep trying to think of what exercises to do.

- **I Don't Have Enough Time**

Who would really agree that they have ever had enough time? No one.

Most people you know, including those ones you see

at the gym or the ones you see jogging each morning or evening, also have chores, school/office work or kids to attend to.

We all do. If the only time of the day to exercise is at 5am, then get up early and make it happen. It's painful at first, but you'll thank yourself afterwards and feel much better for the rest of the day.

- **It Makes Me Hungry**

Exercise is work, so it is logical if you get hungry. You are burning calories. It is advised that you eat a piece of fruit before your workout and make sure to drink plenty of water before, during, and after.

A lot of the time our brain will interpret thirst as hunger, so you think you are hungry, but it's actually your brain telling you need water!

If you are a beginner, this is more of a problem, but over time, the hunger goes away and your body adapts to the loss of calories.

- **My Hard Office Work Is Enough Exercise**

A lot of people are fond of using this line as their favorite excuse when they don't want to get stick to a particular exercise routine. It is all a common excuse to feel better for shying away from a program.

However, this is one of the most difficult excuses to prove wrong because many people are convinced that their job is considered exercise.

Many people are really convinced and it becomes a big excuse for them to skip their program.

The only way your job counts as exercise is if you are an exercise instructor, a personal trainer who works out with his or her clients, or any other fitness-related job that involves sweating.

Even if you wear an odometer at work and find out you are walking 4 miles each day on the job, it counts as activity, not exercise. There is a big difference between the two.

As we step into a new week, get back your mojo again. Pick up your trainers, your dress and whatever materials you use and get back to work.

You can still have that shape you wanted because other did same thing and got same results.

Remember that those who succeeded gave no excuses.

How to Handle This Fat

You can tone your belly by abdominal exercises and other exercises we have talked about.

Brisk walking daily or alternate days, as your time permits is recommended.

Jog for about one and half hours at a time (about 75 minutes). Add some vigorous or power exercises like lift up, sit up, pushups and squats.

Also, a change in your diet is also important. Eat a healthy diet. Emphasize plant-based foods, such as fruits, vegetables and whole grains, and choose lean sources of protein and low-fat dairy products.

Limit added sugar and saturated fat, which is found in meat and high-fat dairy products, such as cheese and butter. Choose moderate amounts of monounsaturated and polyunsaturated fats — found in fish, nuts and certain vegetable oils — instead.

Replace sugary beverages. Drink water or beverages with artificial sweetener instead. Water still is the best.

Check the size of food you eat at each sitting. At home, reduce your portion sizes. It's time to stop loading your plate like a mountain as you used to do.

In restaurants, you can share meals, or simply order half portion (half plate).

Remember that you're not doing this because you cannot afford the food but because you want to help yourself and live healthier and happier.

In addition, strength training exercises are recommended at least twice a week.

If you want to lose weight or meet specific fitness goals, you might need to exercise more.

In order to lose that excess fat and also prevent it from returning, you should continue your exercises and keep watching what you eat.

Keep active and be focused on what you want to achieve. Aim to lose at least one kilograms in a week. If you can do that, won't you be happy with what you can do in two months?

You'll be doing fine.

Belly Fat and Weight Loss

We learn every day. We develop daily too, in many ways. And you will always challenge each time you that our brains have unlimited capacity for knowledge of which we use only a little fraction during our life time.

Yes, Even if you lived to be 85 or 100, you only used a small part of that power no matter how active it was!

This knowledge made me to truly believe that nothing is impossible, if one could imagine it. But imagination only without a backup action, doesn't achieve anything.

That corresponding action is where you may have been failing. As a superpower that you are, you are never short of ideas. Big beautiful ideas. You only lack the will to step in and that is where you will have to work on yourself.

Any good intention needs a step taken to make it work. It must not be very big steps at the beginning. Just few but consistent steps as you progress, and success would be achieved.

The truth is that once you believe it in your mind, that everything is possible. All of history and human civilization have proven this to us times without number. It is a truth.

Dealing With Your Big Belly?

We know that many people dislike a fat and protruding tummy. Millions hate it.

Millions of us prefer the flat, firm abdomen, the type that allows you to wear the kind of shirts, blouses, trousers and skirts you like.

A big belly is a "show spoiler" for many people as you can no more buy some type of clothes no matter how you like it and even if you have the money.

It makes it difficult for you to zip up your fine jeans.

It makes it difficult for your belt to look smart and "show face", even if it's a designer belt, the bulging tummy sometimes overlaps and folds it in and you just feel like cutting off that portion, if it were possible.

Have you seen such before?

Not many people like to have such annoying, wobbly fat hanging down their front.

However, it's also true that our bodies tend to store fat

more around the waist as we get older. This seems to happen more in women than in men but men also have same problems.

An expanding waistline is sometimes considered the price of getting older. For women, this can be especially true after menopause, when body fat tends to shift to the abdomen.

The main issue with this belly fat isn't just because of all those the things that were mentioned above. No.

The most important concern is that it carries significant health risks that should bother you.

However, you shouldn't be too scared because the threats posed by belly fat can be reduced or altogether prevented.

How Do People Get Belly Fat?

It is a surety that you'd like to know why people develop this bulging tummy in the first place so that you can know what to do.

Isn't that your thought now?

Our weight is mostly determined by two causes:

- Our diet: That is how much we eat and

- The activities we get ourselves engaged in or, how active we are.

Body type and hormones also play their own roles.

If you exercise a little and eat much (living a sedentary lifestyle), you're sure to add fats to your abdominal region, including in your belly. Some of your friends may be telling you that you're now "enjoying" but, in truth, you're becoming unhealthier.

Ironically true.

Also, as we age we lose muscle mass and fat increases. Muscles help in burning away fat and you can see why as some people get older, they tend to grow fatter and this can affect attempts in losing weight.

The likelihood to add weight around the abdomen — will lead you to having an "apple" shaped abdomen instead of the desirable "pear" shape abdomen — genetic factors are also implicative.

The issue with fat in the belly is that it's not just about that bulge we all see and talk about. (Subcutaneous fat). Belly fat also features visceral fat. This type of fat is deeply positioned within the abdomen, neighboring some vital internal organs.

Even though subcutaneous fat that sometimes leads to some cosmetic issues, visceral fat on its own is connected with far more risky health challenges, such as:

- Type 2 diabetes

- Heart disease

- Breathing problems.

- High blood pressure

- Abnormal cholesterol

Research has also has linked abdominal fat with a heightened risk of developing cardiovascular disease. You can see why we talk about carrying too much fat in the tummy.

CHAPTER THREE
DIET AND WEIGHT LOSS

Metabolism

When we were younger, we loved big vocabularies. High sounding words or convoluted sentences. It made us feel "big". We somehow respected those who could so speak and all the senior prefects who sprayed their sentences with some uncommon words. We were awed each time a teacher used some big words in class and we'd usually, afterwards rush to our dictionaries to know what the meaning was. The few students who could buy some novels usually threw up some big words extracted from the novels and made us envious. The senior students, especially the "Functionaries" as they were called would memorize some big words or sentences and assemble us for some "important announcement" where they simply barked some stale instructions which main but, veiled purpose was to display their newly acquired knowledge.

We were still impressed because we were entertained in such a manner except when some bullies among them sent their sticks crashing on our backs and butts for their pleasure and, "respect".

There are many high sounding words used by people in certain industries which confuses those outside and the weight loss industry isn't an exception.

The word metabolism may sound common to you but to some, it's another big word which makes them think that they might not be getting something correctly.

Does Metabolism Affect Weight Loss Or Gain And Can It Be Increased Or Decreased?

Anyone who's interested in his/her weight control must have heard many times and many things about metabolism, both the truths and the junk.

Metabolism simply means the series of chemical reactions in a living organism that create and break down energy necessary for life.

In a simpler term, it means the process by which your body works to convert whatever you eat or drink into energy for other activities.

Does Metabolism Make You Lose Weight?

The reason some people think this way is, they believe that burning of calories more than one consumes, will make one to lose weight. And, yes. They are correct. That's actually how it works.

It is also true as said above that, metabolism burns calories hence they think that increasing the metabolism will also increase the calories burning, hence accelerating weight loss.

Sometimes we even read about certain things to take to speed up metabolism. Is it really true or possible?

Even though you cannot control your metabolic speed and functions, you have much control over the amount of calories you that your body burn by regulating the level of your activities.

That's the much you can do.

Fact is that the more active you're, the more calories you burn. And that burning and presentation of energy for your body use as you engage in activities is called metabolism.

Does it make any sense now?

Sometimes, certain writers especially in this weight control industry, speak of metabolism as if it's a magic wand that makes all excess weight to disappear by revving up your body functions like it were brand new automobile.

It doesn't work that way.

The best way to shed excess weight or to prevent acquiring it is to regulate intake and to increase physical activities to enable you balance your calorie intake and energy expenditure.

Change Your Diet

It is true that there is currently no best diet or set of dietary instructions for handling thyroid-related issues, but then, making some significant changes in your eating habits is very crucial in helping you get rid of unnecessary weight.

The type of dietary scheme you stick to, however, is a function of your exclusive physiology, ability to absorb food nutrients, food sensitivities and allergies, and the effectiveness of your body at metabolizing, storing, and metabolizing carbohydrates. The idea is to consider the different means of achieving a fit and trim physique, and closely stick to the object of your research.

You may also consider…

Cutting You Daily Calories Consumption Levels

You may like to check the label on your groceries to ascertain the calorie levels in the foods and drinks that you consume. There is also applications that can help you calculate the amount of calories that you are consuming. Get them installed on your phone and proceed to calculating the calorie levels in your foods.

Increase Your Fiber Intake

Getting a good amount of fiber is one of the basic tactics you can employ as a thyroid patient if you want to lose weight. It can come from high-fiber foods, supplements, or both. One great tactics that you employ to help you shed off some annoying fats is to include high amount of fiber in your diets and cutting shot the levels of carbohydrates that you consume: Typically diets that have a low glycemic index would do.

The Paleo diet

A whole foods diet, low-sugar, unprocessed, the Paleo diet, can reduce inflammation. Just make sure you're getting enough iodine.

A low carbs diet: These diets are characterized by a very low carbohydrate nutritional value. Examples of these types of diets include the Atkins and the famous Ketogenic diet.

- **Changing Your Meals Timings**

You may like to practice intermittent fasting diet as a mini solution to weight loss. Limiting the frequency at which you consume to two or three meals everyday with no other food and no snacks after 8 p.m. is effective in stimulating the process of fat break down, and also help regulate the activities of hunger stimulating hormones.

- **Get Tested For Food Allergens**

Prevalent allergens like soy, wheat, dairy, and certain nuts and fruits may also be implicated in fat accumulation. Try eliminating any of these allergies from your diet if you are suffering from their effects.

A Gluten-free Diet

There's a connection between celiac disease and gluten sensitivity and the commencement of autoimmune diseases, such as Hashimoto's thyroiditis. Engaging in a gluten-free diet can lead to a significant weight loss. Certain studies in some patients have suggested these facts.

Discipline yourself to engage in this diet for a period of three months. If during this period you seem to notice that your energy levels have increased, plus you also experience some significant drop in your body fat and less bloating, then this is an indication that excluding it would help you lose weight.

Proteins

Aside the significance of fatty foods during the course of weight loss, foods that have a high protein content also have their consequences. For anyone who wants to lose weight or reduce belly fat, protein intake is important. In fact, it has a natural property that makes it seem like magic but, it's simply the way it works.

Protein is an important food group in our diets. It provides the building blocks, called amino acids, for the body to be able to renew and repair cells, heal wounds and produce many of the chemicals and hormones the body needs to function.

There is lots of scientific evidence that shows protein is an extremely important contributor in any weight loss program.

Some studies suggest that increasing the amount of protein you eat is the absolute best thing you can change in your diet to achieve weight loss.

How does protein do that?

Eating more protein can reduce craving for other food, potentially reducing calorie intake. It can also boost metabolism, which means the body uses up more calories, leaving fewer calories available to be turned into stored.

You would also have noticed that eating good foods that are rich in protein in the mornings would keep you feeling full during the day and this fullness keeps you from snacking(usually on junk foods), thereby keeping your weight under control.

It helps burn excess calories and hence, keeping fat away from your midsection.

Belly fat 'finds its levels' and you'd be getting as trim and fit as you wanted. Of course, you need to combine it with the exercises as we have been talking about.

Some research has shown a link between protein and belly fat. Many studies have observed that the more protein in the diet, the less belly fat people have.

Much of the research about protein and belly fat suggests that protein intake should account for around 30% of total calories

How Do You Get This Protein?

Foods such as meat, chicken and fish are well-known sources of protein. Other great sources of protein are eggs, seafood, nuts and some whole grains, legumes - for example, peas, beans, groundnuts, melon – and dairy products.

As a matter of fact, melon stands at 23.4% in the plant protein category, making it comparable to other plant proteins food sources such as soybean.

Boost your protein intake by eating more especially

the ones that are readily available in our environment, and are affordable also.

It is good to get your protein from a variety of different sources on a regular basis.

With a generous intake of the regular proteins you already know and combined with the exercises. Just as we have implied earlier, you can touch your body shape in an amazing way. It doesn't have to be expensive and too difficult.

Plant Based Foods

Humans are best suited to consume plant-based foods, irrespective of what is taught in schools or what food producers propagate.

Even Nutritionists and Physicians err in this regard too, well, they can't be blamed.

When wrong knowledge has been so taught and indoctrinated into people in a particular space, it becomes native, and is upheld as the truth.

All the same, we can unlearn whatever we've wrongly believed, and change our practices to align with our new gained knowledge and truth.

For this reason, you should endeavor that your foods are essentially plant-based, centering primarily on vegetables and fruits, then grains, pulses, nuts and other plant foods.

Plant-based foods, primarily vegetables and fruits, are not only the foundation of a healthy diet, but also the best kept secret of successful weight loss.

This is because they can easily fill you up without giving you much calories.

While most refined foods contain a lot of calories in just small portions, vegetables and fruits are just the opposite.

You can eat them generously while consuming fewer calories and yet feel full at the end of your meal.

The Amazing Benefits of Onions

As kids, we anticipated that sizzling sound and the aroma that announced that something good was happening in the kitchen whenever those chopped onions crashed into the hot vegetable oil.

Then, as they tumbled and danced around in the oil, they are soon followed by the tomato paste, then fish or meat, then the spoon that stirs to arrange them accordingly.

In that order.

It is almost a certainty that everyone reading this book must have shed tears because they sliced the onion.

Have you wondered why it even makes people cry?

Why Eat Onions?

Eating vegetables of all kinds helps to reduce the risk of many lifestyle related diseases. Onion is a big member of the vegetables and herbs family which help in this fight.

Onions are part of a family of vegetables and herbs known as allium. In this family is also the garlic, chives, leeks, scallion etc.

The onion contains vitamins A, B6, C and E. Onion is a good source of folic acid too. It also has minerals such as sodium, potassium, iron and dietary fiber.

Many of the foods in the allium family have been associated with the prevention of cancer, especially stomach and colorectal cancers, prostate cancer, and

50

esophagus cancer.

Extensive researches on the causes and prevention of some cancers have proven that the allium vegetables can inhibit unnecessary growth and also prevent the formation of free radicals.

Skin Health

Because onions are high in vitamin C which is needed in maintaining the collagen, it helps to keep the hair and skin healthy. Collagen helps you look young, your skin, smooth and free of wrinkles.

It keeps your hair full and prevents thinning and falling off. It keeps your hair fresh and growing well.

Phytochemicals

Phytochemicals are very important class of food nutrients because of their unique role in building the body's immune system and spearheading many other important physiological processes. They help to fight cell death which in turn makes you not only healthier but younger also.

Onions contain them and together with the Vitamin C, they boost your immunity.

So, get it generously present in your next meal. Try not to throw it away from your grilled meat and other foods you usually found them in.

Do not bother much about the bad breath it gives immediately especially if you're going to be in a group conversation.

Plant foods help to promote weight loss, a bright healthful complexion, hair, increased energy and overall health.

The truth is that this is bigger than having a momentary breath which you can handle well with mints and a good mouth wash.

Let the benefits be your motivation and your lesson. Continue to eat healthy. Be mindful or deliberate about what you eat.

Drinking Water and Weight Gain

Here are a few salient points to note

Water contains zero Calories. And so ultimately does not promote weight gain. However, when you do drink a lot of water and climb on the scales, yes the scales will reflect that you have gulped a gallon. But make no mistake about it, when you eventually empty your bladder you will pass out most of it.

Water can promote weight loss and is highly recommended in your weight loss regimen or to use as such, drink at least one glass full before meals, it will take up food space....so you won't "over-eat' and "over-add".

Other Benefits of Water Intake

- It helps in BP control

- It promotes a Clear face

- Water improves digestion and detoxification.

- Water can dissolve kidney stones too.

And lots more...

CHAPTER FOUR
LIFESTYLE AND WEIGHT GAIN

The Doctor Who Defeated Obesity by Overcoming His Addiction for Food

While the reason for the obesity of others was the result of a congenital disorder, it wasn't the case of Kevin Gendreau. This 31-years old medical doctor contended with an unpleasing addiction for food for many years. At his heaviest, he was weighing an incredible 301 pounds. This is enormous for the type of lifestyle he intends to lead.

"I was diagnosed with high cholesterol, hypertension, high blood pressure, sleep apnea, and fatty liver disease, and some things diseases," Gendreau said. "It was obvious that my eating habits triggered all of these, but surprisingly, I couldn't help it."

He turning point and wake-up call when his biological sister came down with terminal cancer. Ever since then, it was his sole mandate to make his health his priority. "While she was suffering from the consequence of what was not exactly the result of her actions," he said. "Mine was a different ball game. It was all my fault. My eating habits."

By taking out the junks from my food and replacing them with vegetables, fruits, protein, and nuts, He was able to shed off 125 pounds in just 18 months.

"Finding the courage and motivation to orchestrate a change is one of the best advice I can render to anyone out there who wants to give weight loss," he said. "The eye opener for he was when I discovered that my sister needs to be there for her kids, but wouldn't because of her. Your motivation and drive could stem from something else. When it comes, be courageous enough to make a good use of it. When your decision is within the confines of reason and common sense, commit to it. This is your shot, you sure don't want to lose it."

How Sleep Can Cause Obesity

It is actually scientifically proven. Yes. Recent studies linked sleep duration and weight gain. But the burning question remains how?

In one of the studies done by experts on weight loss,

constant sleep deprivation in men increased their demand for high calorie foods, which affected the overall calorie intake.

It also suggested that women who slept more than nine hours each night or less than five hours were more likely to gain about five kilograms.

The hormones in the body are said to be responsible. They are called Ghrelin and Leptin.

It was also suggested that lack of sleep led to fatigue and fatigue can make one to be less active.

Sleep deprivation sparks a cycle that always slow your metabolism, lacking energy and keep you feel tired.

It messes with your hormones too and all these can lead to adding that excess weight you have been avoiding.

This should be another reason for you to take that rest in the day and grab a sound sleep at night.

It is not a question that regular exercise promotes better sleep. When you engage in regular physical activity, it can help you fall asleep faster, get better sleep and deepen your sleep.

Just don't exercise too close to bedtime, or you may be too energized to go to sleep.

Working From Home and Weight Gain

A lot of us who work from home can look like we're having the time of our lives by others who don't.

People think you get to wake up whenever you want, work whenever you want and do whatever you like.

While working from home has its merits like not having a regimented time for work, no traffic to and from work, no paying for an office and increasing your business expenses, there are a lot of draw backs as well.

If you get to work from home, you find that you get to work longer hours than if you were at an office. You can work 12 - 18 hour days.

If you work from home, you most likely have no social life, as opposed to popular belief. This is because you get to a point where you can't tell where your work stops and life begins.

You work eventually becomes your life. All you talk about when you eventually meet people, is work. You spend weekdays and weekends working. You get so tired that you'd rather sleep than go out or hang out with friends.

You can develop work-related health issues like fatigue, insomnia from turning your bed to your office, stress from working constantly, and most commonly, aching back and shoulders from not having a proper seating chair and table.

You are usually hunched over your phone and laptop on a chair or on the bed for hours on end. You develop poor posture and constant aches and pains in different parts of your body that no one can understand where they come from.

You will develop poor eyesight over time from working under terrible light conditions and the constant glare from your phone and laptop screens. You find yourself skipping meals and being constantly dehydrated, leading to loss or gain in weight, depending on your body type.

You get frequent headaches that may develop into migraines from the stress, fatigue, eye strain, poor posture, terrible diet and dehydration.

The result of all these is that you find yourself constantly sick, with monthly episodes that last longer each time and become more difficult to treat. These are known facts because a lot of people have experienced them first hand.

How Can You Manage to Survive This?

You can start be developing a system to take care of yourself and even though it may initially seem that you are not very good at following your own rules, you'll quickly realize that when you do, you will certainly feel a lot better. This may be the magic moment that you have been waiting for. To make the most of, you need that dedicated focus and persistence to make it count.

There are lots of coaches and books out there that will teach you how to work from home and avoid falling into the pit of work-related health issues, particularly weight gain and possible, obesity.

CHAPTER FIVE
BEATING NATURE OWN'S FORCES

The Woman Who Wouldn't Be Stopped By Her Thyroid Condition

When nature gets in the way, life can sometimes be a bed of roses or a thorn in the flesh. And when it is a thorn in the flesh, only a miracle disguised as the laws of science may proffer solutions. Such is the case of Desiree Alexis-Kae Mize, an eight year old child that was diagnosed with a congenital condition known as hypothyroidism.

This condition is one of the prevalent congenital conditions that affect Americans. To put in perspective, there are more than three million American with this aberration. One of the most prominent symptom of this disease is the fact that whoever has it also have a slower rate of metabolic reaction.

When Desiree gets engaged in activities that help increase the pace of her metabolism, she would temporarily lose some weight. But in the long run, she would always get those weight back. Sometimes, the regain comes in greater proportion than it should be. When she turned 21, she was weighing a whopping 260 lb. something that made her feel less of herself, and more probe to the actions of bullies. To make her have a positive outlook on life and remain socially active, her doctor recommended that she undergo gastric bypass surgery. This would help her in getting rid of some of the fats that accumulates in her gastric region to so that she would be fit and trim.

Desiree intuitively knew that the gastric bypass surgery done would be her best option, but her resolve to get the surgery done at all costs became even greater when she heard of the exciting success stories of obese people who have undergone the procedure and have their lives changed in the process.

Quoting her by her own words "it became obvious that portion control would be possible with the help of surgery, but then, I'll have to discipline myself throughout my entire existence to keep myself fit and healthy". The truth is that when the desire to lose weight is mixed with discipline and commitment just like Desiree foretold, weight loss would become a tangible reality.

Exactly one year after the surgery was done on Desiree, she lost about 150 pounds. To make this new found joy an enduring reality, she maintained a lifestyle of continuous exercise and healthy eating. It is true that the ball got rolling because a doctor performed a surgery on her, but it became her sole responsibility to make sure that that none of those annoying fats ever make it so her system again, at least to her gastric region.

"I feel like I'm finally confident and happy with my body and myself," she said. "It is true that gastric bypass surgery is not the best choice out there, but then, I have already decided that it was what I needed because I knew that it was the right choice for me, and as luck would have it, it worked for me. I do not only get to see seemingly impossible results as a result of my congenital condition—but I have also become stronger healthier by watching out for my weight."

How to Lose Weight if You Have a Congenital Thyroid Disorder

For a lot of people, the act of weight loss can be a very frustrating and tiring process when they have an underlying thyroid abnormality. Whether your thyroid is removed due to surgery or you have hypothyroidism, it is not a question that your metabolism is affected by the presence or absence of the biochemical produced by the thyroid glands.

Below are some stunning tips that can be of help to you in your quest to dealing with the frustrations that comes with the desire to lose weight, as well as some of the secrets and common dietary schemes that you can engage in to make this a feasible reality for you.

Quickly Get Diagnosed

An insufficient treatment or a total lack of it for an underactive thyroid is a recipe for an impossible weight loss scheme despite the engagement in exercise and diet. When diagnosis is prolonged, the tendency to keep gaining weight would only skyrocket.

While you are turning hypothyroid, and your TSH (Thyroid Stimulating Hormone) levels suggests that you seek treatment, there would be a significant slowdown in your metabolism, meaning that you'll only get to lose an insufficient amount of calories. This condition that can also lead to situations of tiredness, and a lack of desire to engage in an exercise program. This would even serve to further decrease your metabolism. Your body is wired in such a way that when you are fatigued, there would be a growing tendency in you to foods containing high amount carbohydrates so that you can be enriched with the required energy levels to keep you active.

Consult the services of your health practitioner if you have symptoms of hypothyroidism so that you can be properly diagnosed and have treatment commenced on you

Managing Your Weight When You Have Hypothyroidism

Consider Optimal Treatment

When dealing with weight loss, general good health and relief of symptoms is not enough for your doctor to give you a prescription after diagnosis. Also, there is a need of optimal treatment to make sure that your body cells have the required amount of energy and oxygen that they would require to keep the metabolic process going.

When these symptoms persists, then do not relent in discussing with your doctor or health practitioner about the treatment procedure that you may undergoing. If your health practitioner is insistent on maintaining the normal physiological status quo due to some reasons that you do not fully understand, then you should consider seeking for a second opinion, probably from another health practitioner or even a specialist.

Some Useful Medications to Treat Your Thyroid Disease

Test Your Hormone Levels

And since it has been demonstrated that hypothyroidism and hyperthyroidism have the ability to create insulin resistance, you may also like to get your insulin and fasting glucose levels tested, estimated, and treated if necessary.

Studies have consistently shown that issues regarding

hormone resistance – like insulin resistance and leptin resistance – are major key players in the difficulties that people face when they want to shed off some weight.

Your fasting glucose levels can exceed 100, and when this happens, it may be an indication of pre-diabetes and insulin resistance, and these can even make weight loss more difficult.

Drugs like Glucophage (metformin) may be prescribed by your doctor when it is obvious that you have type 2 diabetes. For borderline levels of these endogenous indicators, decreasing the carbohydrate and sugar levels in your diet while sticking to a wholesome carbohydrate-controlled diet can help you decrease the sugar levels in your blood and hence, you can shed off some weight.

Carefully Consider the Treatment Options For Hyperthyroid

You should carefully consider if you need a RAI against other hyperthyroidism treatments. It is common to gain weight after RAI (Radioactive Iodine). A popular study on patients that underwent a thyroidectomy discovered that those whose first line of treatment was surgery were less likely to gain weight or become obese than the folks whose first line of treatment was RAI. You may also like to have a discussion with your doctor about other treatment options that you must have read on the internet.

You should also have it at the back of your mind that patients that underwent a thyroidectomy, the surgical removal of the thyroid, or the RAI treatment have later come down with hypothyroidism.

Have a plan in place with your physician for regular thyroid testing after surgery or RAI so that your treatment can start as soon as there is evidence that you are hypothyroid. Also, your body may experience a delay in the production of the needed biochemical between the period when you first got your treatment and the period when you get a replacement therapy for your hormone levels.

Nutritional Options for Thyroid-Friendly Diets

- **Hydrate**

When you take more water, it helps your body metabolism to be more efficient in its operation. It would also help you in the elimination of bloating, decreasing your appetite, and also improve your digestion and elimination.

The truth is that this is no small advice. When you prioritize the practice of drinking 8 ounces of water every day, you'll notice significant changes in your body size.

In fact, a lot of experts in the industry recommends the habit of drinking an ounce of water for every pound of scale weight. This may be a great deal for most people. But the truth remains that if you have the desire to shed some weight, then you have no option than to do it.

Practice Metabolism-Friendly Exercises

For a lot of thyroid patients, a diet overhaul or even calorie restriction is not sufficient to let for weight loss. Your metabolism can be lowered Hypothyroidism, this means that you only require smaller amounts of calories. This makes it increasingly difficult to decrease the sufficient amount of calories you require to produce appreciable weight loss.

One vital thing to do to enable you raise your metabolism is the fine art of engaging in exercise programs. Your metabolism and general endogenous calories and fat burning processes becomes more efficient when you work out, also your blood sugar levels would be reduced.

If your aim is to lose weight, the exercising more would help you achieve quick and desirable results.

In accordance to CDCs (Centers for Disease Control and Prevention), people of average weight will require about 75 minutes of intensive activity or 150 minutes of modest physical activity every half a month in order to keep to a healthy weight and prevent excessive weight gain.

If want to lose weight and you're hypothyroid, more than an hour of exercise every day is needed to keep you fit and trim.

If you have to prioritize which type of exercise to do, consider strength training and exercise that builds muscle for the maximum metabolic benefits.

Familiarize Yourself with Your Medications

A lot of the drugs that doctors prescribe for their patients who have thyroid-related conditions or other issues you could have been the reason why they even added weight in the first place. The following medications, for instance, are linked with weight gain:

Antithyroid drugs like PTU (propylthiouracil) and Tapazole (methimazole), used to treat hyperthyroidism and Graves' disease

Beta-blockers, such as Corgard (nadolol), Tenormin (atenolol), and Sectral (acebutolol), are frequently used in the treatment of hyperthyroidism.

Steroid anti-inflammatories like progesterone and prednisone Estrogen, either together or alone in hormone replacement therapy or in hormonal birth control

Also some antidepressants like Zoloft (sertraline), Paxil (paroxetine), and Prozac (fluoxetine) are helpful treatment option.

Anticonvulsant and mood-stabilizing drugs such as Tegretol (carbamazepine), and Depakote (valproate)

would also go a long way.

If you're gaining weight even after taking any of these medications, it is in your best interest to talk to your doctor and relate your findings to him. Do not for any reason quit taking your meds without the input of your doctor.

Some health experts and nutritionists have suggested that you ditch your morning exercise and rather utilize the time to find some good sleep. Target about seven hours or more to sleep for every night if weight loss is a challenge.

CHAPTER SIX
MEDITATION AND YOGA PRACTICES FOR PEOPLE WHO MUST LOSE WEIGHT

When you try out your long desired weight loss fantasy, it is almost not a question if you'll be frustrated or of you'll run out of patience. In fact, the truth is that when you are just starting out, you are most likely going to be wary and frustrated about it. The practice of weight loss is not as forthright as calculating your amount of calories you consume and the amount of calories your burn out. There are several scientific studies that suggest that the practice of counting calories is utterly ineffective, in fact some experts discard it as a myth and old-fashioned. Let's redirect our focus and plunge into meditation and yoga as an effective method of losing weight!

There are plethora of factors that leads to weight gain. Most of these factors are very much dependent on our lifestyles and habits. Although some genetic consequence can also be the reason why people add weight. For example, when you do not consume food the right food and in the appropriate proportions, weight gain and eventually obesity may set in. Some bizarre and seemingly inconsistent factors like stress can also lead to weight gain.

Lots of research and documentations have suggested that the degree of stress that we face and the psychological effects they have on us can lead to the addition of fat. This is because stress can increase the catalytic ability of certain stress hormones whose actions can have help increase the amount of endogenous insulin in the body.

This process is one of the numerous processes out there that can immediately and significantly alter the composition of the body by decreasing the body's muscle mass and increasing body fat. When dealing with obesity that sprang up from the activities of hormones, you can be eating food that have a balanced nutrition and still end up adding weight.

Yoga and meditation can be your savior if your weight gain is the resultant effects of stress. When you meditate, your body would be strength it needs to fight stress and when it does that, cortisol, which is chief hormone that induces stress would have its activity reduced. With its level in the blood decreased, the body would start decreasing the levels of insulin and hence also shed off some unnecessary fats that it accumulated. The end result is that the person would become fit and trim in no time.

Just as meditation is an excellent weight loss solution, yoga is also good at it. Even though the practice of yoga may not directly instigate processes that'll burn lots of fats, the consequence of some of its practices such as *"pranayama"* (the practice of breathing) are predominantly advantageous in helping the body burn excess calories. By comparison, the calorie density of lipids is more than that of carbohydrates and proteins and hence hey need a tangible amount of oxygen to metabolize them and release the energy that they the body will need. When you start perfecting the practice of *"pranayama",* your lungs would have increased ability to contain larger volume of air, meaning that your body would have greater volume of oxygen which can facilitate the metabolism of these excess fats and hence, weight loss.

Also, the duo of meditation and yoga are also helpful when dealing with eating to compensate for certain emotional traumas. When you eat, your body will usually release a biochemical known as endomorphin. Endomorphins are implicated in mood change, so that they can make you happier. This can make you more addicted to food and cause weight gain in the long run. This is the reason why food can trigger a knee-jerk mechanism that is helpful in coping with stress. Meditation and yoga have also been implicated with improving well-being and helpful alternatives to fight against weight gain that is due to emotional eating.

If you are adding weight as a result of stress, or maybe you have opted for different dietary regimens and still find it difficult to shed some of those annoying fats, then you may like to try out the meditation and yoga solution.

Also, have a consistent timing that you do this. One effective way of making it with this solution is to practice it about three time every week. You can start it first thing in the morning as a way of relieving you of any lingering stress and making your mind free and prepared for the day's activities. What you are essentially doing is that you are rewiring your brain and mind for a successful tour for the day.

To benefit from yoga breathing, you will need to perform two deep breathing sessions per week. Give it a try and please do share your results!

Also, you may like to carry out two deep breathing activities every week. Try it out. The result will astound you!

www.ingramcontent.com/pod-product-compliance
Lightning Source LLC
Chambersburg PA
CBHW050654250726
48662CB00002B/676